The New Doctor

Romances for Seniors

seniorality

The New Doctor -
Jamie Stonebridge, Stacy J Roberts

Copyright © 2024
Seniorality / Everbreeze Media Oy

This is a work of fiction. Names and characters are the product of the author's imagination and any resemblance to actual persons, living or dead, is entirely coincidental.

Set in 22 pt EB Garamond

Chapter 1
A Hectic Day

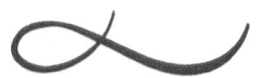

MOLLY JACOBS pulled into her usual parking spot, grabbed her purse, locked the door to her car and dashed into the health center.

"Morning Pearl," she called to the receptionist while hurrying past.

The middle-aged woman waved from behind the desk and continued with her phone conversation. Molly rushed through to the staff area at the rear of the building and placed her things in her locker, smoothing down her uniform before beginning her shift.

She had slept through her alarm and her cat, Blade, finally woke her with a gentle tap on the nose. She hated to be late, scolding herself as she looked at her computer.

Molly scrolled through the list of morning patients. Looking up at the wall clock, she realized that she had ten minutes before her first appointment.

"Just enough time to grab myself a coffee," she grinned.

Chloe was already in the canteen, hugging a mug of the hot brew. Molly smiled at her best friend as she got her own drink, although she frowned when she asked, "I thought it was your day off?"

"It's meant to be, but my cover called in sick," Chloe groaned.

Joining her at the small round table, Molly sympathized as she sat down. They had dreamed of becoming nurses since they were little girls growing up together, but they had both discovered that the hours could be really tiring.

Wimberley was a small town and its number of residents still hadn't reached the three thousand mark. With its natural beauty and with all the activities on offer, more and more tourists were coming to visit the town.

With that in mind, the health center opened a walk-in clinic for those who were hurt or feeling unwell while on vacation in Wimberley. This meant that their workload had increased, leaving their boss with no option but to advertise for another doctor to join the practice.

As the surgery doors opened, Molly returned to her assigned examination room. She was soon engrossed in her work, taking blood samples, dressing wounds and giving jabs to the constant flow of patients she tended.

Between appointments, Molly joined Chloe, helping with injuries that tourists had suffered on hikes or random accidents when out in the street.

She was relieved when the health center finally closed at the end of the day. Feeling exhausted, she splashed some cold water on her face in the ladies' room.

Looking at her reflection in the mirror, Molly could see the dark circles begin to form beneath her eyes.

"You really need to get some sleep, girl," she chuckled to herself.

But she knew that wouldn't be happening any time soon. She had already arranged to go for drinks with Chloe after work. After freshening up, she met her friend in the car park.

The two women linked arms, taking the short walk into the town square.

"O'Neil's Bar?" Chloe asked as they strolled down the main boardwalk.

"Definitely," Molly agreed.

Kris O'Neil's wine bar had become one of their favorite haunts when Molly and Chloe were downtown. Their preferred bottle of wine was quickly placed on the bar as soon as they walked through the door.

"You know just what we need, don't you, Kris?" Molly purred as she slid onto a stool.

"I am always ready for you, beautiful ladies."

The two women laughed as they took a welcome drink from the glasses he poured. Kris was known for his flirting, so they rarely took his comments seriously. Molly still couldn't help admiring his good looks.

He was a tall man with a shock of brown hair and deep chocolate eyes that twinkled when he spoke. His skin was deeply tanned and his toned muscles were always on show in the tight-fitting tops he wore.

However, his handsomeness didn't change the fact that he was considered a womanizer, someone Molly didn't want to get involved with. Yet the flirting they shared when she went to the bar nevertheless excited her.

Now, as Kris moved on to serve other waiting customers, Molly turned to her friend and asked, "How are you enjoying living in Paradise Hills then?"

"I truly can't believe that I inherited the place!" Chloe gasped. "I mean, I knew I had an eccentric Aunt who hadn't married, but I never imagined that she would leave me her house."

"She must have loved you very much," Molly remarked.

Chloe's expression turned somber as she recalled some painful memories. "My parents tried so hard to help her over the years. I can remember visiting the house when I was younger. In the end, she barely knew who we were."

"That must have been so upsetting," Molly said, gently touching her friend's hand.

"It was, but the fact that she left the house to me makes me feel so lucky and grateful," Chloe admitted.

For the next couple of hours, the friends chatted happily, refilling their glasses before ordering another bottle.

Wimberley was like a forgotten town hidden in the High Country of Texas. It was nestled along the banks of Cypress Creek, which ran into the Blanco River. However, the most prestigious place to live was Paradise Hills.

There, homes had been built into the rock side, providing owners with stunning views across the landscape. Only those with money could afford the expensive price tag to live in such a stunning place.

"You deserve it," Molly soothed.

"Felix and I have moved in, but it just feels so strange to be there without my aunt sitting in her usual armchair," Chloe confided.

"I can imagine, but, I am sure you will be happy there," Molly reassured her.

Chloe suddenly took Molly's hand, eyes wide as she suggested, "Why don't you come over this weekend? We can have a barbecue in the backyard."

Once they had agreed on a time, Chloe called her husband to pick her up. Molly booked a cab home a few moments later.

Yet, before she had a chance to leave, Kris caught Molly's arm.

"Wait, please," he said.

Molly could hear the sincerity in the man's voice as he continued, "I was just wondering if I could take you out for dinner one night?"

Suprised by the invitation, Molly held her calm when answering.

"That sounds lovely, but we are rather busy at the health center just now. So I'm not sure when I will next be free."

As she climbed into her cab, Molly looked back and saw the disappointment on Kris's face. She hoped that she had let him down gently as she was driven back to Woodcreek.

Arriving outside her house, she paid the driver before going inside. Still with Kris on her mind, her thoughts raced as she changed into a short pink satin nightgown.

She wasn't sure if dating someone like Kris would be such a good idea. Yes, he had money and was clearly intelligent enough to run a successful business. However, he also came with a lot of what some might call "baggage," and she knew better than to trust an attractive man with many women at his beck and call.

She had been hurt some years earlier when an ex-boyfriend cheated on her. She wasn't keen to experience that feeling ever again. Yet she knew what Chloe and her husband would say.

They were always telling Molly to stop overthinking things. To just go out and have some fun for a change. As well as being very easy on the eye, she knew that she would have a good night with Kris.

Although, she still faced a dilemma. "I'm getting too old for the partying and late nights. All I want is a nice guy who I can cuddle with on the couch while watching a movie. That isn't something I could imagine Kris doing," she thought to herself.

Her cat Blade jumped onto Molly's lap as she sipped from a glass of wine she had poured. Absentmindedly, she stroked his soft black fur, his purrs growing louder as he curled up.

When she first brought the kitten home a year ago, he was just a little ball of fluff. Since then, he had followed her everywhere, always there to give her cuddles whenever she needed them.

"What do you think I should do, Blade?" she asked the cat.

He only softly meowed his reply, causing Molly to smile down at her pet lovingly. The night was beginning to draw in, the outside lights on her patio starting to shine amongst the flowers and greenery.

When she first visited the one-bedroom property, she had been captivated. Not only was the house itself beautiful, the views across Cypress Creek were also breathtaking.

Now, the water's colors were beginning to darken as the sun sank lower in the night sky. The leaves of the nearby trees were a deep green and wafted in the light breeze, which helped cool the warm air.

Due to the local public course, Woodcreek was popular with retirees and golf enthusiasts. So Molly had found living there to be relatively peaceful, which she appreciated after a hard day's work.

Tonight was just as serene as always, only the late calls of birds before they settled into their nests could be heard.

Blade objected grumpily when Molly stood up before quietly, sliding the floor-to-ceiling windows closed.

"Sorry, darling, but it's getting late. I've got work in the morning, so it's sleep time."

With that, Molly turned off all the lights and crawled under her covers, slowly drifting off into a restful sleep while Blade settled beside her.

Chapter 2
A Strange Meeting

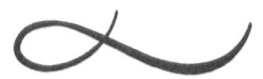

MOLLY SET off on her walk to work early the following morning. As always, she enjoyed her leisurely stroll along the banks of the creek toward town. During these times, she appreciated the peace of her surroundings.

Now, all she could hear was sweet birdsong from the trees that towered overhead. Lush green grasses ran alongside the path she followed, while blankets of aromatic flowers danced in the breeze.

The sound of traffic grew louder as she approached the busy main street. Wimberley was now considered a resort town, attracting many tourists who enjoyed its natural beauty.

Along the main street were original limestone buildings, each store with its own brightly colored timber façade. All the streets in town stretched out from the central square, a place where local events were held, like markets and concerts profiling up-and-coming bands.

Cypress Creek ran through the square before flowing into the Blanco River further downstream. The tall cypress trees that ran along the water's bank gave off a pleasing aroma. It was a refreshing smell that reminded Molly of pine and seemed soothing somehow.

The young woman had spent many of her lunchtimes sitting amongst their thick roots, breathing in the enchanting scents, which provided an air of tranquility. A contrast to the hustle and bustle on the streets just yards away.

When Molly reached her favorite diner, she pushed open the door. Immediately, she inhaled all the tempting aromas drifting through from the kitchen.

Despite it still being early, Brown's Burger and Grill was already crowded. George, the owner, was busy cooking while his son, Davey, worked alongside him. A bell rang when each plate was ready to be served.

Finding an empty booth in the far corner, she scanned the menu.

"Morning, Molly, what would you like?" Rosie, George's daughter and waitress, greeted her with a pad and pen poised, ready to scribble down her order.

Usually, Rosie was full of vibrancy. She was a twenty-three-year-old with a curvy figure who always revealed a little of her ample bust. All the customers adored her as she dashed between tables, always with a smile.

But today, Molly noticed how tired her friend looked. Her face was pale, and her blonde curls were already hanging loose from their clips. The normal spark in Rosie's sky-blue eyes had dimmed.

With concern, Molly touched Rosie's hand gently and asked, "Are you all right?"

"Every table has been full since six o'clock this morning. My feet are killing me already," she grumbled.

"Have you had the chance for a break?"

Rosie rolled her eyes, and Molly's heart went out to the young woman. The whole family was committed to the business. Their hours were long, allowing little time for themselves.

So, while the waitress plated her order, Molly sneaked behind the counter. Hiding her personal things before serving a large mug of sweetened black coffee. Plating a warmed croissant and bagel, knowing they were all Rosie's favorites.

"Molly! What are you doing," Rosie gasped.

"Serving you breakfast for a change," she grinned.

When she saw the appreciation on her face, Molly knew that she had done the right thing. Tying an apron around her waist, she approached a family who were just sitting down, leaving her friend to tuck into her food hungrily, murmuring with delight at the taste of the freshly baked pastries.

Once Rosie had eaten and she had finished her own meal, Molly quickly ate hers before pecking her friend on the cheek and calling out a cheery farewell as she dashed back into the street. Time was ticking, and the health center would be opening soon. Desperate not to be late, Molly quickened her pace but abruptly stopped when she saw a man ahead of her sitting on the ground and clutching his ankle.

"Are you okay?" she asked politely.

"Yes, I'm fine," the stranger answered with a grimace.

Yet, when she looked at him, Molly felt something surprising. Her eyes were transfixed on his as she tried to catch her breath. She couldn't explain it, but she felt such a powerful attraction to this person she had never met before.

"Please, I'm a nurse at the local health clinic, let me help you."

However, she was stunned when the man suddenly began to chuckle.

A frown deepened on her brow while she waited for him to explain. "Well, this wasn't exactly how I intended to introduce myself. But I'm Steve Henderson. The new doctor at the surgery."

"Wow! I can't believe it! It's a pleasure to meet you," Molly gasped.

She shook his hand vigorously, her mind racing as she scolded herself…

"Come on, Molly, the man is in pain here. Ignore the nerves, pull yourself together, and get him some help!" she thought to herself.

She gently placed an arm around his waist, helping him to walk while he groaned in pain.

"Let's get you to the clinic and check that ankle out," Molly said, her voice reassuring.

With each arduous step, the man winced. However, he didn't complain as they slowly walked toward the health center.

He was panting as he asked, "So, could I ask the name of my rescuer?"

"Oh, I'm sorry," she blushed. "I'm Molly Jacobs, one of the nurses."

As soon as she indicated towards her uniform, she immediately chided herself silently, realizing that as a doctor he would surely know how to recognize a nurse's uniform.

It was time for her to get a grip, before she made a fool of herself, she felt.

"Well, I owe you my thanks, Molly. Although this certainly is not how I wanted to begin my first day."

"I bet," she laughed.

She instantly regretted her laughter. Lowering her gaze as she mumbled, "Please accept my apology, Doctor Henderson. It was rude and thoughtless of me to laugh like that."

Coming to a stop, he turned her to face him. His eyes shone like jewels of jade.

But his words sounded earnest as he told her, "Don't apologize; you have done nothing wrong. It was my own silly fault for not watching where I was going. And please, only call me Doctor Henderson when we are in front of a patient. Otherwise, it's Steve."

They exchanged a gentle smile and Molly felt her stomach begin to flutter nervously. She pushed aside the feeling as they continued on their way. Molly gave him a sideways glance as she asked, "So, Steve, how did you twist your ankle exactly?"

Molly had stressed his name intentionally, hoping to put him at ease. His smile told her that the plan had worked as he explained, "All I did was go into the Deli to pick something up for my lunch. Although, I must admit that I wasn't looking where I was going when I came back out. Too busy checking my phone."

She caught his sheepish expression before she quipped, "Ah, the curse of today's technology."

"Hey, stop teasing - I already feel terrible," he joked. "You see, the next thing I hear is a dog whimper and then I got this little old lady trying to beat me with her cane. She was yelling at me and saying I stood on her dog's paw."

"I was so shocked that I staggered backward and fell off the curb. I landed on my behind, but because I hurt my ankle, it took me and age to get back on the sidewalk. The woman just left me there."

Unable to stop herself, Molly burst into giggles, waving her free hand to try and excuse her reaction.

"I'm sorry, Steve, but I wish I had seen that. It sounds like you have met Mrs. Wilson. She is something of a character around Wimberley and a regular at the health center. The old dear is also very protective of her dog."

"Oh great, what a way to meet one of your patients," Steve groaned.

"Don't worry, I'm sure you will win her round."

By now, they had reached the health center, although Molly was disappointed that their conversation was coming to an end. Pearl must have seen them approach as she was ready to open the door and a wheelchair was waiting for them. Molly helped Steve lower himself into the seat of the wheelchair. As soon as he was comfortable, she steered him to their small X-ray room.

"You go and catch your breath before the first patients arrive. I will take over here." said one of the other doctors.

"Thank you, Walter." said Molly.

Doctor Walter Farrington had been the trusted physician for numerous families in Wimberley over the years. He was a tall, slender man who was now fifty-six years old.

Yet, despite him being happily married for the past twenty-three years, women still swooned over the silver-haired man.

Walter had employed Molly five years ago, and they had grown close over that time. Molly nodded her thanks again before disappearing into the staff rooms at the rear of the clinic.

Chloe waited for her in the canteen, holding out a mug of coffee. She took it gratefully before slumping into one of the worn armchairs.

"The day hasn't even started and I already feel exhausted," Molly chuckled.

Her friend sighed heavily in exasperation before pleading, "Never mind that! What is he like?"

"Who?"

"The new doctor, of course!"

"Oh, you mean Steve."

While Chloe's jaw fell open in disbelief, Molly shrugged casually, a broad grin on her face as she thought to herself…

"You really shouldn't tease her like that!"

But they had been inseparable since childhood, so she knew Chloe wouldn't truly believe her fib.

"That's just what he wants to be called unless there is a patient around, of course."

"Why do I get the feeling you have taken a liking to him?" Chloe said knowingly.

"Don't be silly." frowned Molly unconvincingly.

However, as the young nurse continued with her morning, the new doctor never seemed to be far from her mind.

Chapter 3
A Walk-In Wonder

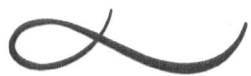

MOLLY HAD left the car at the health center last night in anticipation of her morning visits. So, with her case filled with medical files, she drove off to see her patients. When she returned to the health center at lunchtime, her stomach was grumbling hungrily.

Pearl sat in the canteen, tucking into a prawn salad that she had brought from home. She was a small, plump, African-American woman with a strong, yet compassionate personality.

On one hand, the forty-nine-year-old could be as gentle as a tiny kitten. But if you annoyed or angered her or threatened anyone she loved - then, she became like a lioness protecting her cubs.

Molly pulled up a chair opposite the receptionist and opened a container of pasta with shredded beef drizzled with a mild mustard dressing.

Before Molly could take a bite, Chloe joined them. When she saw her friend's expression, she knew she had something to say.

"So, Pearl, what do you think of our new doctor?"

With a raucous laugh that echoed around the room, Pearl declared, "Now, if I weren't a married woman, that man would definitely be on my radar."

"And I think our Molly feels the same way," Chloe teased.

However, before Molly could object, they all fell quiet when Walter and Steve strolled into the room. The young doctor was thankful to slide onto an empty chair after limping across to the table.

Walter stood beside them all, clearing his throat, "Well, I was going to make the introductions this morning. But it seems some of you have already met. Even so, I would still like to welcome Steve Henderson as our new doctor. I'm sure you ladies will all make him feel at home and a part of our little family."

Pearl was already making a fuss, fetching Steve a cushion to rest his ankle. The others just exchanged polite smiles and murmured a brief greeting. Molly was secretly hoping that she would have the chance to get to know this curious stranger better.

She was able to disguise her delight when Walter announced, "Molly, I want you to help Steve today, please."

"Certainly," she answered casually.

However, Chloe was far from fooled when she caught up with her friend a few moments later.

"You got a lucky break there, didn't you," she said with a wink.

"I don't know what you mean." replied Molly.

Molly tried to remain nonchalant but couldn't look her best friend in the eye for long. Eventually relenting with a heavy sigh before saying, "Okay, I admit it; I'm happy that we have been paired together for the day. But it's not as if I can really get to know him during the walk-in clinic."

"Ah, but you will be able to watch his muscles flex as he works."

"Stop teasing me!" Molly whispered, feeling her cheeks flush.

"I'm sorry, I won't say anything else," Chloe put up her hands in defeat. "I will leave you to your day with the handsome doctor."

While Chloe went to meet her first patient after blowing Molly a kiss, Molly rolled her eyes before going through to the clinic area.

The two girls had first met in pre-kindergarten when they were just three years old and they have been close ever since. Often getting caught by the teachers or their parents when they got into mischief together.

Chloe was more like a sister and Molly couldn't imagine life without her.

"It's just a shame sometimes that we know each other so well. These days, I can't get away with anything as she always seems to predict what I'm thinking," she sighed, though her warm grin remained.

A couple of patients were already seated in the walk-in clinic when Molly strolled through the large swing doors. One was a stranger, but the other was a local and the nurse immediately went to her.

"Tracy, I didn't expect to see you this morning. What's wrong?"

As the young woman burst into tears, Molly ushered her through to an examination room. Tracy Burns was only nineteen and had given birth to a baby girl just six months earlier.

Her long brown hair appeared unbrushed this morning, hanging loosely to her shoulders. Anxious brown eyes darted back and forth, as if she was unsure if she should be there.

Molly offered her a seat, where Tracy settled while nestling her daughter close. Molly waited while the young mom gathered herself, dabbing her eyes with a tissue before she could speak.

"Can you check Tiffany for me, please? I don't know what's wrong, but I have been up all night with her. She wouldn't stop crying and nothing I tried quietened her."

"Of course, I will," Molly said as she took the small child.

While examining her, Tiffany gurgled happily. She was the image of her mother, with the same deep brown eyes and small tufts of light mousy-colored hair that were already beginning to show on her scalp.

Molly had visited the new mom numerous times and she and the baby were both doing fine. The nurse could easily see how much Tracy loved her daughter; all she needed was a little confidence that she was doing a good job.

Now, as she looked at the woman, her expression was gentle and understanding. Her voice was soothing as she told her, "Tracy, Tiffany is fine. But you look exhausted, and she will sense that. Is there no one that could help? Just so you could have a break for a couple of hours."

And as soon as Tracy lowered her head, the nurse scolded herself. Molly had forgotten that Tracy had no family that she could turn to.

"Listen," Molly soothed, "I have a friend who runs one of the local mother and baby groups. I'll give her a call, so she can welcome you to their next meeting at the local civic center."

"Really?" Tracy gasped.

"Yes, and you can hear the other mothers' stories while you're there. Perhaps you might believe me then when I say that you are doing great Tracy. I know that you need some sleep but give this group a chance. I'm sure you will make some solid new friends who will help support you."

"Thank you so much," the woman gushed.

"It's my pleasure. You and this little one deserve to be happy. But you also need to know that you are not alone."

Grinning broadly, Tracy took her daughter with an air of contentment that Molly had never felt in her before.

"That young lady is going to be just fine," she told herself confidently as she watched her leave.

"Very nicely handled."

Spinning around, she found Steve leaning against the wall. His face was caring, as he strolled closer, perching on the edge of her desk.

"Referring her to your friend like that was such a thoughtful thing you did for her."

"Well, I just think it would be helpful for her. Tracy is a wonderful young woman, but she needs to have more faith in herself."

"You are a very caring person, Molly. I haven't seen a lot of that lately, so I'm finding it quite refreshing."

"I guess that's how things are in towns like Wimberley. We all look out for one another here."

"That's exactly why I decided to buy into the practice. I got so fed up with working for large private clinics. I wanted that community feeling in my life again."

"So, you grew up in a small town, too?" Molly queried.

"Yes, much like this place. It's something that I have been missing and, surprisingly, I have felt more at peace since moving here."

"You're planning to settle in Wimberley long term, then?" Molly's heart beat a little faster, waiting to hear his answer.

"Oh, I'm aiming to stay here for keeps," Steve beamed.

While a feeling of relief washed over her, she had little time to ask more. The whimpering cries of a little girl spurred them both into action. A middle-aged bearded man carrying the child, yelled out desperately, "Please! Can someone help my daughter!"

"Bring her through here," Steve urged the anxious father.

Quickly following, it was clear that the girl had broken her ankle. After an x-ray to confirm the diagnosis, a cast was fitted. Even though she was now calm and comfortable, she pouted as she stared at her leg.

"What's wrong, sweetheart?" her father asked.

She eyed him sadly and innocently replied, "I'm so silly, falling over like that."

Steve's sudden outburst of laughter made everyone in the room stare. Although the tiny patient was soon joining in when he told her the story of his first morning at the medical center.

Showing her his own ankle support and x-rays while she looked at her dad and said, "Perhaps I'm not the only silly one after all."

Watching Steve with the little girl showed Molly a tender side to the new doctor. She was hopeful that she would soon see more of this handsome man.

Chapter 4
A Girl's Night Out

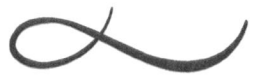

WHEN FRIDAY night rolled around, Molly was eager to meet up with her best friend Chloe. They got together at the end of each week. Molly hoped for a couple of hours dancing to blow away the cobwebs.

Since their first encounter, Steve had been constantly on her mind. Every time she saw the doctor, her heart began to race. Occasionally, their hands would touch accidentally, sending a surge of electricity running through her body.

The young nurse was confused by the strength of her feelings. She had never experienced such an intense attraction before.

Molly chose a little black dress that clung to her hourglass figure. She slipped into some smart heels, picked up her bag and dashed from the house. Her cab was in the drive, patiently waiting with the engine running. She slid onto the backseat and a short time later, she was joining her friend outside the nightclub.

It wasn't long before the women were inside. They soon weaved their way through the throng of people to order drinks, having to shout over the loud music so the barman could hear them. There was little chance of conversation, so they took their glasses of wine onto the dance floor, moving their bodies in rhythm to the music.

The club was crammed with early evening partygoers, and everyone seemed to be absorbing the mood after a busy week at work. Molly finally began to relax in the vibrant atmosphere. It didn't seem long before she needed to order fresh drinks from the bar.

"Are you trying to get me drunk?" Chloe giggled.

"Don't be silly. I'm just in the mood to have some fun," Molly declared.

Another tune began and a crowd surged toward the stage. This time, the two friends merely watched, only rejoining the other dancers when the floor had cleared a little.

Molly was soon lost in the music and her own thoughts, moving to the beat as if she were the only one there. Her legs and arms began to warm as the time slipped by as she danced. She was jolted back to reality when she felt a hand on her arm and saw Chloe motioning to her.

Over the years, the girls had created a secret code that only they understood. Chloe used it now to indicate that she was hungry. Molly nodded to agree as they maneuvered toward the exit. The doorman gave them a cheery farewell as they left the club. Chloe linked arms with her friend as they strolled down the main street.

"Sorry for dragging you out of there, but I'm hungry."

"No problem, me too."

After some discussion, they opted for the Chinese restaurant nearby. A waitress led them to an empty table and served them water while they ordered.

Leaning across the table, and speaking in a whisper, Chloe asked curiously, "Molly, you really like Steve, don't you?"

"Yes, I do. But that is hardly the point." said Molly.

"What do you mean," her friend frowned, not understanding Molly's almost defensive reply.

"Look, it doesn't matter how I feel about Steve" added Molly. "He is not only a colleague, but also my boss, so it would be wrong.

Chloe's expression was one of disbelief as she pointed out, "Who cares about rules Molly, if this is your chance to find love?"

"It doesn't matter anyway. I mean, there is no guarantee that Steve even feels the same way."

"Bet I can get him to talk," Chloe winked.

"Please, don't!" pleaded Molly.

"Ok, ok. I just hate that you won't take a chance every now and again. Just because your ex cheated on you, doesn't mean that all guys will do the same. You have to learn to trust again."

Molly knew that Chloe was right, but it was something that she couldn't face right now. Everything that her ex put her through had caused her a lot of emotional pain. She had never imagined being with anyone else since then. Yet, Steve had stirred feelings in her that she simply couldn't explain.

Plates of food were placed before them, which they both began eating eagerly. The tang of spice caught her tongue, but not to be distracted, Molly could see that there was still something on her friend's mind.

"Do you think if Steve were interested, you would get involved?" Chloe probed.

"After the stuff I've been through... men are not my priority. If it's meant to be, then God will allow it to happen." replied Molly.

Since splitting from her last boyfriend, Molly had enjoyed being single. True, she missed the hugs and spending time with him each day, but at least now she could again be the person she once was. After spending two years under his influence, Molly enjoyed finally being able to make her own choices in life again. She was determined that she would never be manipulated like that again.

"He is nice, though, isn't he?" questioned Chloe.

Molly nodded, unable to disagree. Although they had only worked with the new doctor for the past week, Steve had certainly proven popular with patients and staff alike. Steve Henderson was a kind, thoughtful, and polite man who always seemed to appear just when he was needed – as if by magic. He was witty and often had people laughing at his comments.

But most of all, the doctor possessed a certain unexplainable air that made people feel instantly comfortable around him, easing any nerves so they were confident enough to confide in him.

Molly found him easy to talk to and enjoyed their conversations when they worked a shift together. They spoke between seeing patients, and she soon discovered that they had many of the same interests. Both enjoyed reading and watching movies while sharing a passion for keeping fit. Molly felt like she could chat with him for hours.

"So, what's Felix up to tonight?"

"Quick change of subject," Chloe said laughing at her friend's obvious attempt to avoid talking about Steve anymore. Chloe answered, "He's over at the pool hall with his friends. Apparently, some qualifying matches are being played."

"Well then, let's finish up here and get over there to cheer him on," Molly said with a grin.

"Are you sure? I didn't mention it because I didn't know if you would be in the mood," Chloe admitted.

"Don't be silly; I would be happy to go and watch them play."

After they had eaten, the two women paid the bill and headed down the street. Their heels clicked on the sidewalk, as the friends walked arm in arm.

The music from the nightclub was a faint memory as they neared the pool hall. Pushing the heavy glass doors open, they could hear the potting of balls on the nearby tables. Two matches were being played, and the women waved when they spotted Felix waiting to take his shot. They ordered drinks from the bar and settled in some chairs that gave them a good view of the game.

However, they both sighed heavily when they saw who Felix's opponent was. Kris O'Neil, one of the best pool players in the whole county. Yet, they crossed their fingers, hopeful that Felix might still be able to win. Tension mounted as each ball was potted in turn and Molly couldn't tear her eyes away from the table. Behind her, she heard the drone of the other spectators, all giving their hushed opinions on the next best shot.

As Felix potted the black, a cheer erupted. The large bell behind the bar rang as more drinks were ordered to celebrate his win. Chloe leapt from her stool and raced to her husband, throwing her arms around his neck. Leaving Molly smiling to see her excitement and the love the couple obviously shared.

"I wouldn't mind a hug of commiseration."

Molly flipped her head around at the sound of the voice. Kris stood behind her, a cheeky grin on his face.

"I don't think so," she answered, shaking her head.

"Oh, come on! I mean, it is your fault that I lost."

Kris sat beside her, taking a gulp of his beer before placing the glass down.

"What?" exclaimed Molly!

She was confused. What could she have possibly done to cause him to lose? She eyed him incredulously, waiting for an explanation.

"You see, I was distracted as soon as I saw you. Your beauty shone so brightly; it was all I could think about."

Her sudden burst of laughter shocked some people, who glanced with wonder. Molly politely but firmly told him, "Listen, there might be some women out there who will believe it when you say things like that. Sadly, for you I'm not one of them. So please, stop wasting your breath, Kris; I'm truly not interested."

When she saw the hurt flash across his eyes, Molly felt a pang of guilt for her bluntness. She was surprised then when Kris gently took her hand, and spoke earnestly, "Sorry, Molly, I never meant to hurt or upset you. I will respect your wishes and leave you alone. But what I said about your beauty was true. I just hope that the man who catches your heart sees it as clearly as I do."

Feeling a surprising tenderness toward the bar owner, Molly kissed his cheek lightly. They clinked their glasses together in a sense of friendship as they all enjoyed the rest of the evening.

Chapter 5
Accidents and Attractions

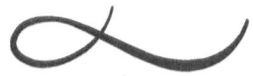

THE FOLLOWING week, Molly was busy taking stock of the supply cupboards at the health center. However, she stopped with her pen mid-air when she heard raised voices in reception.

"I've told you! I need to see someone now," a voice roared.

Racing through to the main entrance, Molly stopped in her tracks. A tall, muscular man was towering over Pearl, an angry glare in his eyes. The older woman held her ground as she rose to her feet. She looked small beside him, but her no-nonsense tone spoke volumes as she told the stranger, "Now you listen to me, young man, that attitude is unacceptable in this health center. So, you can either have a seat over there and wait for the next available nurse, or you can take your bad-mouthed backside somewhere else."

The man sat down with a sheepish expression. Molly gave her friend a secret nod of approval from where she hid in the doorway, emerging despite the remaining tension in the air.

"Good morning, sir; how can I help you today?" Molly addressed him boldly.

When the stranger raised his face to her, the nurse immediately sympathized. There were numerous large red blotches on his skin, some already bleeding from his scratches. Knowing how frustrating it could be to have an allergic reaction to something, she understood his irritable mood.

From that moment on, Molly's Day passed in a blur. The patients seemed to come through the door as if they were on a conveyor belt.

By the end of the day, Molly was feeling exhausted as she gathered her things from her locker.

Her friend Pearl had already headed home, so Molly turned off all the lights and set the building alarm. She locked the health center doors behind her before crossing toward her car. She was so preoccupied with rummaging through her purse, for her car keys though, that she didn't spot the cyclist suddenly appearing from around the corner of the building.

Molly fell to the ground heavily, landing on her left side. Feeling pain in her arm, she cried out in pain. Her eyes began to well with tears as she started to take deep breaths. A shadow fell over her, blocking the streetlights sun. Davey from Brown's Burger and Grill stared down at her, worry evident in his deep brown eyes.

"Oh my goodness! Molly, are you all right?"

Wincing, she accepted his help to her feet. Yet, she cradled her arm to her chest, suspecting that it might be broken.

"Don't worry, Davey, it wasn't your fault," she assured him.

When Davey realized that she was hurt, the young chef's face paled. He held

Molly to his side as her legs started to weaken, a wave of dizziness washed over her.

Davey wasted no time in calling the emergency services. Molly was helped into the back of the ambulance which took them to the ER at the health center.

She was helped into a wheelchair and taken into center. Moments later, she heard fast running footsteps and then a voice she recognized asking, "Davey, what's happened?"

Steve bent down in front of Molly to ask how she was feeling before she was taken into a cubicle. Molly felt quite embarrassed as various colleagues popped in to check on her, before Doctor Walter came in to check her out and organize x-rays and scans.

Molly had fractured her left arm and had been badly bruised when she fell. Her arm was put in a cast and the doctor said that she must stay in overnight for observation.

Steve popped in to see her once she was settled in a room and gave her two featherlight kisses on her cheek. He asked if she would like to give him her door keys so that he could pop in and feed Blade when he finished work.

Molly fell asleep and was vaguely aware of nurses popping into the room regularly to check her. Late the next morning, Doctor Walter said she could leave the Health Center and go home where she should rest as she would be on sick leave for the next week.

She was pleased to be back at home and Blade was certainly very happy to see her too. Having had a broken night's sleep, Molly decided that a short nap in her own bed would be perfect.

Snuggled under the covers, Molly fell asleep quickly. She woke some hours later to the sound of television faintly in the background.

Gripped with apprehension, she padded barefoot into the lounge, hovering unseen, among the shadows, nervous about what she would find. She soon relaxed when she saw Steve lounging on the couch, Blade curled up beside him. Molly couldn't help but smile when she heard the doctor talking with her cat about the program being shown on the screen.

"Well, this certainly wasn't something that I thought I would wake up to," Molly laughed as she stepped into the room.

Steve jumped from his seat, struggling with his words as he stammered, "I, erm, didn't hear you come, er, come in."

"So I saw, the pair of you were really engrossed," Molly said, motioning to the cat.

Sitting at Steve's side, she could sense his nerves. She remained casual as she motioned toward the open carton of chocolate milk at his side.

"Could I have a glass?"

His broad smile showed his mischievous side as he gave her a cheeky wink.

"Now, let me think. I mean, you have sustained quite an injury."

"Oh, stop it!" said Molly.

Playfully, Molly slapped Steve on the arm. But inside her stomach were butterflies fluttering frantically.

"Thank you for bringing me home and staying with me," she smiled.

"I couldn't very well leave a damsel in distress," he quipped in reply. "I got hold of Chloe who met me at the Emergency Room. It was her idea to use your spare key and bring you home. She's quite the friend to you. She just left maybe 30 minutes ago."

"I just hope that Davey doesn't feel too bad about it. It was just an accident at the end of the day. I should have looked before stepping out."

"Davey is fine; now stop worrying and just relax. Doctor's orders!"

Reluctantly, she nodded, accepting her drink. Changing the subject, Molly commented casually, "You certainly seemed to have made an impression on Blade."

The cat was now settled on the back of the couch, his eyes flitting between the pair as if he were listening.

"He has made an impression on me, and certainly helped to keep me company while you rested in the other room."

Later after they talked a while, and she thanked him again, Molly was left feeling disappointed when Steve headed home. She locked the door behind him.

Still feeling weak Molly got comfortable on the couch to watch a movie that had begun to play and slowly fell asleep. However, some hours later, the sound of loud knocking woke her. Molly opened her eyes to find sunlight streaming through the windows. Nothing but static showed on the television screen, and she quickly turned it off.

Glancing at the clock on her stove, she was surprised to discover that it was already lunchtime. Her grumbling stomach confirmed the late hour as she opened the front door. Steve stood on the step, a wicker basket in his hand.

Although her brow creased in confusion, Molly couldn't help her smile at seeing him again.

"I thought I should come and check on my patient and make sure she has eaten."

"That is so kind of you," said Molly smiling.

Steve strode through to the kitchen as she closed the front door behind him. Blade followed quickly on his heels, immediately smelling the warm chicken.

"Don't you worry, Blade, I haven't forgotten about you," Steve informed him.

"Really? You have even thought about Blade!" she gasped in disbelief.

"How could I not? He's part of your family, he's your companion and best friend."

Until now, only Chloe had understood Molly's attachment to Blade, understanding the comfort that he brought her since she had moved into a place on her own.

Yet, when she looked into Steve's eyes, she knew that he also realized just how much she loved her cat. Blade now happily rubbing against his new friend while purring loudly.

Steve dished up the sumptuous food on two plates: rice, vegetables, and thin slices of roast chicken. He even served some for Blade in his cat bowl so he could tuck in alongside them as they ate.

"This is delicious," Molly said through a mouthful of food.

"My mother's recipe," Steve admitted.

She eyed him teasingly as she asked, "So, who actually cooked this? You, or your Mom?"

"Hey, this effort is all mine," Steve threw up his hands in his defense, "It would taste ten times better if my Mama had made it."

"Sorry, I shouldn't have tormented you."

"There is no need to apologize, Molly."

For a while, they fell into silence. However, from the corner of her eye, she could see that he was deep in thought as he sat there. Finally, he spoke, "Hopefully, you might get to meet my parents one day soon."

Before she could comment on the idea, he hastily changed the subject. Molly wondered if perhaps he regretted the suggestion when she saw his flushed cheeks, remarking instead how strange it would be on Monday morning without her at the surgery.

"Don't worry, I don't plan to be off sick for long."

Steve smiled but then eyed her seriously, saying, "No, Molly, I won't allow it. You can't come back to work until you are fully fit."

Reluctantly, the nurse had to be sensible and agree. Especially considering the strength of the painkillers she had been prescribed. Even now, her eyes were growing heavy once more.

Leaving Steve to load the dishes into the dishwasher, Molly thanked him and they then said their goodbyes as she needed to rest.

Resting her head on her bedroom pillow while Blade curled up close by, Molly nestled down with a contented smile. She remembered the moment Steve had gently kissed her brow as he left.

That night that she slept soundly. Visions of the handsome doctor filled her mind as she imagined a future with the pair of them together.

Chapter 6
A Romantic Date

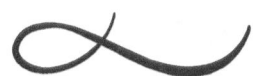

THE NEXT morning, Molly woke to the smell of freshly brewed coffee. Warily, she crept from her bedroom. Her heart beat rapidly, wondering how she could possibly have slept through the noise if intruders had broken in.

She sighed with relief when she saw Chloe in the kitchen, pleased to see her good friend, who had used her spare key to open the front door.

"What time is it, Chloe?" Molly sounded surprised.

Chloe turned to face her, a smile on her lips as she chuckled, "It's eleven o'clock in the morning, sleepy head. How are you feeling today?"

"Goodness, I can't believe how much I'm sleeping!" Molly gasped.

"Make the most of the chance to rest and having Steve look after you," Chloe advised her with a big grin.

Chloe then suggested that Molly should relax all day as Steve would be popping by after to work to check on her and Chloe knew for a fact that he wanted to invite Molly out for dinner two evenings later – if she felt well enough.

Molly, looked down at the crumpled nurse's uniform, she was still wearing.

"How could he want to take me out when he's seen me looking like this?"

Chloe said that within a couple of days, Molly would be looking lovely and feeling much better. Chloe said she would come around and help her get ready for her special evening. Chloe then helped to wrap her friends cast in plastic so that she could take a shower to freshen up.

The next two days passed quickly with much of it being spent snoozing on the couch with Blade snuggled in next to her. Chloe popped by during her lunch break each day to see that all was well.

In the evenings, Steve also stopped by after work to see how his patient was doing. On the first evening, he had arrived at her front door with a huge bunch of flowers, which he organized in a large vase for her table. On the second evening, he brought Molly an appetizing selection of fresh fruit.

They agreed on a time for the following evening and Steve said he would not stay any longer as she needed more rest. He got up from the armchair and walked to the couch where he lent down and kissed her gently on both cheeks.

Molly spent the next day once again resting on the couch, with her cat cuddled into her legs. By the afternoon, she was certainly feeling much better.

Chloe came around straight after work and as soon as she saw Molly, declared - "It's pamper session time," steering Molly gently toward the bedroom.

With their favorite radio station playing in the background, the two women rummaged through the wardrobe to find the perfect outfit for Molly to wear, while they sang along to the music.

Once the outfit was decided, Chloe wrapped Molly's cast carefully in plastic so it would not get wet when Molly took a leisurely shower. Chloe was there to assist whenever needed and this included washing her friend's hair.

Chloe blow-dried Molly's hair and styled into waves, with a section secured by a sparkling jeweled clip. Nerves began to flutter in Molly's stomach as she sat patiently while Chloe applied a light layer of makeup. Chloe then helped Molly slip into a thigh-length wine red dress with a daring neckline.

Chloe adorned Molly with a ruby and diamond choker and helped her slip into a pair of comfortable red flats. Chloe had the clever idea of decorating the cast with a pretty silk scarf. Molly grabbed her red purse before checking her reflection in the mirror.

"You look absolutely stunning," Chloe remarked.

"Thanks," Molly replied modestly.

"Come on, let's get you a coffee to calm those nerves."

Back in the kitchen, coffee was brewed, and Molly sipped hers anxiously. She paced around, avoiding sitting down to prevent creasing her dress. Chloe couldn't help but notice her friend's unusual restlessness.

There was a sudden knock at the door, startling Molly. She took a deep breath before answering it.

Steve was wearing tan-colored slacks and a white short-sleeved shirt that was unbuttoned at the collar. His light brown hair was neatly combed, and he beamed broadly as his emerald eyes sparkled.

"Wow! You look truly amazing."

Blushing deeply, she accepted the compliment, along with single red rose he held out.

Chloe waved the pair off, promising to put the rose in water and lock up when she left. Molly gave her a secret crossed fingers signal before following Steve to the cab.

They traveled to the restaurant in silence; Molly wondered whether he was feeling as tongue-tied as she was. So, she welcomed the noise of the restaurant when they finally strolled through the main doors.

The restaurant served French cuisine and was always full. Customers usually needed to make their reservations well in advance to guarantee a table. Tonight, it was their turn to be treated like royalty as the maître welcomed them warmly.

"Doctor Henderson, Miss Jacobs. It is our pleasure to serve you both this evening."

After kissing each of them on the cheek, he clicked his fingers high in the air. Catching the attention of a young waiter who immediately hurried over.

"Take these guests to our finest table in the corner," he ushered.

Following him across the dining room, Molly could feel people's eyes on them. Self-conscious about her arm being in a cast and annoyed with herself for not suggesting another restaurant.

Since moving to Wimberley, she had never dined at this exclusive eatery before. Through her lowered lashes, she spied some of the curious stares that they received.

"What on earth was I thinking agreeing to come here?" she argued internally. "This is the fanciest restaurant in town and I have only one arm in use. How can you possibly think that this is going to end well?"

She smiled warmly at Steve when she sat down opposite him. He must have sensed her unease. Placing his hand gently on her arm to stop her from looking at the leather-bound menu for a moment.

"Are you all right, Molly? You look a little pale."

"I'm fine, it's just a little warm in here," she fibbed.

Glancing around the room, Molly noticed numerous familiar faces. Many of the private patients that she saw at the clinic. They were all giving her a discreet nod of reassurance.

"Why don't I believe you?"

She dared to raise her eyes, seeing Steve's concern as he gazed at her intently. Beams of light from the evening sun fell on him through the window. His caring face seemed to glow beneath its rays.

There was no need for her to speak when he suddenly whispered, "You don't have to worry about a thing; I have connections in the kitchen."

He winked with the same cheeky grin Molly had come to adore. His voice was husky as he leaned closer and explained, "Since moving to Wimberley, I've become good friends with one of the assistant chefs here. So, I had a quiet word before he started his shift, and whatever you order, he will make sure he plates up and makes it easy for you to eat."

Embarrassed by the thought, Molly didn't know how to react. Only relieved when he added with a laugh, "I don't mean making you a shake and serving it with a straw. All he will do is chop the food into smaller pieces in the kitchen so you don't need to struggle with your knife."

Grateful for his consideration, Molly was finally able to relax. She soon found herself absorbed in conversation with Steve that she never wanted to end. Talking to the doctor felt natural and easy, as if the pair had a hidden connection. Something that the young nurse couldn't erase from her mind as the night grew longer.

Although, when they left the restaurant a couple of hours later, Molly was expecting them to hail a cab. Instead,

Steve steered them toward the creek. She offered no objections as they settled beneath one of the cypress trees.

"This place is so beautiful," Molly sighed contentedly.

Steve cupped her cheeks in the palm of his hand, turning her head to face him.

"So are you," he told her.

Barely able to breathe, her heart began to pound hard as his lips drew near. Molly's eyes closed, lost in the intensity of their kiss. She forgot that other couples were also sitting further along the bank, possibly watching them.

When they parted, she could only manage to stammer. "Erm, well, thank you."

"Oh, Molly, you really don't realize, do you?"

Innocently, she shook her head, still unsure what Steve meant. Her stomach began to do somersaults as he gazed at her tenderly.

His hands felt warm to touch as he held hers lightly while saying sincerely, "I have fallen for you, Molly. All I can dream is that you have some feelings for me too."

Her mouth fell open to speak, but she couldn't utter a word, leaving Steve frantically to add, "Listen, I know it might not be ethical because we work together, but I'm willing to resign from the surgery if it means that I can be with you."

"No, you can't do that," she pleaded. "Walter needs you there."

Molly admitted she felt the same way and the pair realized that all they could do was discuss the situation with the senior physician.

They needn't have worried, as Walter was delighted to give them his blessing when they finally spoke to him.

"You are both aware of how to behave in front of the patients. Wimberley is a small town, so word is bound to spread quickly. Personally, I couldn't be happier for the pair of you," he grinned.

He kissed Molly's cheeks and shook Steve's hand firmly before leaving them in the staff canteen.

"Well, that went better than I expected," Steve said, sighing with relief.

"I know, I can't believe it."

Steve wrapped his arms around Molly's waist to pull her closer and their kiss was long and tender before they began their day in the clinic. Both of them were beaming with happiness about the love they had found together.

Epilogue

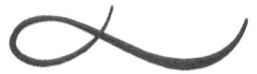

MOLLY JACOBS stepped out of the steaming shower, wrapping a warm towel around her slender frame. Her long blonde locks hung damp against her shoulders as she grabbed another towel to dry them off.

Barefoot, she sauntered into the bedroom, humming along to the song playing on the radio. Taking a seat at her dressing table, she began to run a brush through her hair.

Memories of the past year flooded her mind and she smiled at how much had changed.

When she first laid eyes on Steve, she never could have predicted the impact he would have on her life. There was something about him that drew her to him from the start. Her feelings for him had only deepened over time.

As a couple, Molly and Steve had enjoyed so much together. They frequented the nearby Blue Hole Regional Park for swims and hikes, always packing a wicker hamper full of picnic goodies. They spent evenings at local bars, listening to live bands playing everything from rock to folk and they always moved in perfect sync on the dance floor.

Tonight was special; they were dining at Chloe and Felix's place, a rare gathering of the four friends. Molly looked forward to the evening ahead.

After applying a light layer of makeup, Molly slipped into her favorite blue dress. The strapless number hugged her figure, accentuating her bronzed skin and fell to mid-thigh. She swept her long blonde hair to one side, securing it with a glittery clip.

Choosing black heels and a matching blue purse, Molly blew a kiss to Blade her cat, who playfully lifted his paw in response.

Steve waited in the driveway, and as Molly climbed into the passenger seat, she leaned over to plant a firm kiss on his lips.

"You look absolutely stunning," he whispered tenderly.

"Thanks, handsome," she replied with a playful wink.

He was dressed in sleek black pants and a smart, sky-blue shirt, perfectly complementing her ensemble. She could smell his captivating aftershave, lingering on his smooth skin.

Resting her hand in his, she settled in for the short journey. Despite being a lifelong resident of Wimberley, Molly still found herself awestruck by the ever-changing landscapes.

As they climbed higher into the hills, Molly marveled at the magnificent homes they passed. Though she had visited her best friend many times, each trip felt like entering a whole new world.

Chloe's house, though considered one of the smaller ones on the estate, never failed to evoke a sense of wonder in Molly.

The four-bedroom home was nestled into the hillside, its stark white exterior standing out against the lush greenery that surrounded it. Floor-to-ceiling windows framed in black added to the striking contrast, while the interior was equally impressive.

Felix swung open the large oak front door, grinning broadly as he said, "Head on through to the lounge; Chloe's waiting with drinks."

As soon as they entered the room, a chorus of cheers erupted. Molly and Steve were taken aback by the sea of familiar faces, overwhelmed by the warm congratulations on their anniversary.

Despite the joyous atmosphere, a sense of unease gnawed at Molly. Why all the fuss, she wondered. She glanced at Chloe, who simply shrugged. It wasn't until Steve took her hand that everything began to make sense.

Molly noticed the subtle signal Steve gave to Felix, who promptly raised his arm, signaling for silence. The sudden hush and the weight of all eyes on her and Steve made her heart race.

"We can't thank you enough for organizing this surprise party for us. But I'd like to turn it into a true celebration," Steve announced.

The room filled with tense anticipation as everyone waited for Steve's next words. Molly's nerves intensified as he turned to her, his expression becoming serious.

"It's been a year since we met and I can't imagine my life without you. So I wanted to say something. Something important. Molly, I love you with all my heart and I want to ask if you'll do me the honor of becoming my wife."

Gasps rippled through the crowd as the young doctor dropped to one knee. Molly's mouth fell open in shock, but when she locked eyes with his, she knew her answer.

"Of course, I'd love to marry you!" she exclaimed, delight coursing through her.

Neither of them could believe their luck in finding each other. Molly was overwhelmed with joy, knowing she had found the love of her life.

As Steve slipped the diamond ring onto Molly's finger, the room erupted into cheers and applause. Tears welled up in Molly's eyes as she threw her arms around Steve, feeling overwhelmed with happiness and love.

Amidst the joyous chaos, Chloe appeared at Molly's side, wrapping her in a tight embrace. "I just knew he was going to propose tonight!" she whispered excitedly.

Molly laughed through her tears. It was a moment she would never forget – surrounded by the people she loved, celebrating the beginning of a new chapter in her life with Steve by her side.

Later as they danced together in the center of the room, Molly's heart swelled with gratitude for the unexpected journey that had led her to this moment. She looked into Steve's eyes and knew that their love story was only just beginning.

The End

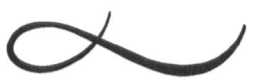

www.ingramcontent.com/pod-product-compliance
Lightning Source LLC
Chambersburg PA
CBHW020435220526
45464CB00002B/722